Using a Brief Intervention to
Motivate Clients to Get Help

Using a Brief Intervention to Motivate Clients to Get Help

A How-to Manual for Professionals

Tracy Stecker, Ph.D.

HAZELDEN®

Hazelden
Center City, Minnesota 55012
hazelden.org

ISBN: 978-1-61649-158-1

Editor's note
The names, details, and circumstances may have been changed to
protect the privacy of those mentioned in this publication.

This publication is not intended as a substitute for the advice of
health care professionals.

Diagram on page 14 adapted from Ajzen, I. 1991. "Theory of Planned
Behavior." *Organizational Behavior and Human Decision Processes*
50:179–211.

14 13 12 11 10   1 2 3 4 5 6

Cover design by David Spohn
Interior design and typesetting by Briana Chapeau

The Dartmouth PRC–Hazelden imprint was formed as a partnership between the Dartmouth Psychiatric Research Center (PRC) and Hazelden Publishing, a division of the Hazelden Foundation—nonprofit leaders in the research and development of evidence-based resources for behavioral health. The internationally recognized Dartmouth PRC staff applies rigorous research protocols to develop effective interventions for practical application in behavioral health settings. Hazelden Publishing is the premier publisher of educational materials and up-to-date information for professionals and consumers in the fields of addiction treatment, prevention, criminal justice, and behavioral health.

Our mission is to create and publish a comprehensive, state-of-the-art line of professional resources—including curricula, books, multimedia tools, and staff-development training materials—to serve professionals treating people with mental health, addiction, and co-occurring disorders at every point along the continuum of care.

For more information about Dartmouth PRC–Hazelden and our collection of professional products, visit the Hazelden Co-occurring Disorders Partnership Web site at www.cooccurring.org.

To those who suffer

Contents

Introduction   1

Program Description   7

Intervention Session Outline

    Part 1:
    The Cognitive-Behavioral Therapy Model   17

    Part 2:
    The Relationship between Beliefs and Behavior   23

    Part 3:
    Alternative Ways to Think   27

Appendices

    A. Solutions for Potential Problems That May
       Arise during the Intervention Session   41

    B. Case Examples   45

    C. PASS Questionnaire   59

    D. iMPASS Questionnaire   67

References   74

About the Author   76

Introduction

Most people with psychiatric or substance use disorders never seek treatment. This unfortunate fact may come as a surprise to many professionals in the mental health and addiction fields. Why a surprise? In part because, of course, mental health and addiction professionals only see those who *do* seek treatment, and they may come to assume that these clients are the most typical. But in reality, in the United States only about one in five people with a substance use problem ever receives professional care. The figure is even lower—one in four—for those with mental health problems. In other words, most people with addictive or mental health problems continue to suffer, even though effective professional help is available.

Of course, getting people into treatment can be difficult. For people with mental health and substance use problems, this may involve extreme measures, such as an involuntary commitment to inpatient hospitalization during an acute crisis. Over the past twenty years, the sources of referral for addiction treatment have shifted. We now see fewer referrals made by doctors and more made by courts and other legal mandates, including driving-related violations. Other approaches have been developed as well. These range from the well-known family interventions for people with substance use problems to contingency management, which involves rewarding those who seek and attend treatment, using vouchers for prizes or other rewards.

Other interventions, such as motivational interviewing (MI), have been developed as well. MI is designed to help an addiction or mental health professional harness the client's own motivation to change. But although MI is effective for helping patients *continue with treatment*, there is no evidence for its effectiveness in getting people *into treatment* in the first place.

Ideally, clients will make that choice themselves. Although mandating or requiring people to enter treatment may provide a nudge for the otherwise resistant client, this external motivation is far from empowering. It risks an oppositional reaction or a superficial compliance. In the best-case scenario, the treatment-forced or externally rewarded client experiences a shift in attitude while in treatment. In these cases, motivation shifts from external to internal. But unfortunately, despite the universal implementation of these forced-treatment approaches, we have scarce evidence for their ultimate effectiveness in changing behavior and improving mental health or substance use outcomes.

It is commonly thought among medical personnel that the main barriers to treatment involve external factors such as cost and travel distance. But evidence has shown that these external factors, although real, do not influence treatment engagement as much as previously thought. In fact, in the well-known Partners in Care study for depression treatment, while 81 percent of patients with depression were referred for psychotherapy in the Quality Improvement (QI-therapy) arm, only 30 percent actually attended a psychotherapy session. That outcome was despite four main advantages for patients: (1) education about psychotherapy; (2) joint treatment decision-making among the patient, nurse specialist, and primary care provider; (3) minimized copayments; and (4) the convenience of psychotherapy sessions offered in the primary care setting (Jaycox 2003). This study convincingly illustrates how few people actually get the treatment they need.

This study convincingly illustrates how few people actually get the treatment they need.

Likewise, in Project iMPACT, only 42 percent of elderly primary care patients participated in psychotherapy despite its availability at no charge in the primary care setting (Unutzer et al. 2002). This fact alone demonstrates that far more is involved in the treatment-seeking decision than issues related to cost and access. One decisive issue often overlooked is stigma. A persistent and pervasive stigma against seeking mental health treatment still exists in our society; and the stigma that clings to mental health and addiction problems plays an important, potentially critical, role in the decision to seek care. As my colleagues and I considered these facts, we appreciated the importance of getting people the

The stigma that clings to mental health and addiction problems plays an important, potentially critical, role in the decision to seek care.

treatment they need, sometimes at all costs. But we also felt that the outcomes would be better and more effective in the long run if clients felt empowered to make the choice themselves. Ideally, clients will act on their own will, in their own best interests, from the very start. In contemplating a different approach to facilitating an intervention, we found cognitive-behavioral therapy (CBT) useful and effective since it has a broad and consistent evidence base—across a variety of disorders and settings—in changing behavior.

CBT has primarily been focused on changing the cognitions and behaviors (and emotions) associated with a client's symptoms and disorders. As such, it has been remarkably and consistently effective on a wide range of problems. But, we noted, CBT had not been applied to clients' beliefs about seeking treatment or help of any kind for their disorders. That seemed to be a promising area since, in our clinical experience, CBT can help clients shift any belief that might lead to problematic emotions and behaviors, so it could be reasonably applied to treatment-seeking behavior as well.

Over the past four years we have been conducting research in applying CBT to promote treatment seeking among persons with a variety of disorders, including depression, post-traumatic stress disorder (PTSD), and substance use. We have drawn on samples of people ranging from military personnel returning from the wars in Iraq and Afghanistan to civilians in hospital emergency departments and primary care offices. We also used media outlets (television, newspapers, and the Craigslist website) to expand our participant base. This manual is the outgrowth of these studies and our direct clinical experience.

It is our intent that this manual be used by addiction and mental health practitioners to help people who need treatment actually choose it themselves. This manual could be equally effective in other settings as well. School counselors could use it as a motivational tool for adolescents, and parole officers could use it to support their clients in seeking evaluation or treatment for possible mental health or substance use disorders. Our goal is to help all people get the care they deserve—and want.

Our goal is to help all people get the care they deserve—and want.

Program Description

In our current culture of quick fixes—fast food, pain relievers, and medications and vaccines to treat and prevent disease—it might seem that the decision to seek help for any kind of suffering would be the easiest decision to make. But among those with substance use and mental health disorders, low treatment rates indicate that the decision to seek help for this type of suffering is *anything but easy*. The decision to seek help for mental health and substance use concerns can be overwhelming, in fact, so overwhelming that most people who need help never even seek help.

This manual presents an evidence-based protocol *to promote the decision to initiate mental health or addiction treatment*. The intervention employs cognitive-behavioral techniques that focus on modifying beliefs about mental health and addiction treatment, so that a client is in a better position to come to a decision about seeking treatment. In one sixty-minute session, a person who receives this intervention can learn to describe and modify his or her negative thoughts and feelings that interfere with coming to a decision about seeking mental health and/or addiction treatment. The general goal of this intervention is to use techniques designed to explore thoughts associated with seeking treatment (such as availability of treatment, roles of patient and care provider, and expectations for outcomes), thus enhancing clients' self-awareness and promoting better, more thoughtful decisions.

In her book *Cognitive Therapy: Basics and Beyond,* Judith Beck outlines ten principles behind cognitive work:

1. It is based on an ever-evolving formulation of the individual and the individual's problems in cognitive terms.

2. It requires a sound therapeutic alliance.

3. It emphasizes collaboration and active participation.

4. It is goal oriented and problem focused.

5. It emphasizes the present.

6. It is educative, aims to teach clients to modify their own behavior, and emphasizes relapse prevention.

7. It is time limited.

8. It is structured.

9. It teaches clients to identify, evaluate, and respond to their own dysfunctional thoughts and beliefs.

10. It uses a variety of techniques to change thinking, mood, and behavior.

While this intervention incorporates many of these cognitive principles and techniques, it is not designed to actually treat mental health or addiction symptoms, nor does it function as a therapy session. Because it is time limited and designed to modify treatment-seeking behavior, rather than function as treatment itself, the intervention does not require an ever-evolving formulation or a sound therapeutic alliance (numbers one and two on the list). It is important for the clinician to differentiate this intervention from a typical cognitive-therapy session. Here, we are focusing not on the symptoms themselves, but on the factors in the client's decision about seeking treatment for those symptoms.

This intervention is not designed to actually treat symptoms, nor does it function as a therapy session.

The Intervention Session Setting

The intervention session can be delivered by phone or face-to-face. Delivering it by phone may benefit those who are resistant to mental health and/or addiction treatment, or are otherwise unlikely to schedule a face-to-face appointment (perhaps because of geography or transportation issues). This intervention session may be the person's first mental health or addiction treatment experience. As such, it may provide them with a better understanding of the treatment process, especially for those who have inaccurate or incomplete perceptions about it. Receiving this intervention by phone would be an important first step for this type of treatment-resistant person. On the down side, using the phone, the clinician lacks access to certain dynamics that would be present in a face-to-face session, such as body language. Moreover, a client in need of alcohol treatment could even be drinking during the phone intervention session. So, if working by phone, the clinician might need to explain a few requirements at the beginning of the session: find a place with few distractions, do not drink during the session, and so on.

Delivering the intervention in person can be done in a variety of settings, including primary care offices and mental health or addiction care facilities. The intervention is also applicable within the military system, schools, and the criminal justice system as well. It can also be done in a group setting, but even in a group, each participant will process his or her own beliefs individually.

Administering the Intervention

The intervention lasts approximately forty-five to sixty minutes and should be administered by a trained clinician with experience in cognitive-behavioral techniques. Some clinicians may need additional supervision during initial sessions. The chart on the next page shows the session structure, and how the time can be distributed and focused.

This intervention session may be the person's first mental health or addiction treatment experience.

The intervention lasts approximately forty-five to sixty minutes.

Structure of the session	
Introduction Parts 1 and 2 Describe the cognitive-behavioral approach and answer questions.	5 minutes
Elicit Beliefs about Treatment Part 3 Examine accuracy of beliefs and develop alternative thoughts (optional: use PASS or iMPASS Questionnaire).	35 to 50 minutes
Wrap-Up Summarize, reflect on next steps, and make referral if necessary.	5 minutes

Assessing Beliefs about Treatment

Two questionnaires can be used to assess the client's frequently endorsed beliefs about mental health and addiction treatment. The Perceptions about Services Scale (PASS) is for those with mental health concerns, and the Modifying Perceptions about Services Scale (iMPASS) focuses on beliefs about addiction treatment. Both measures are found on the program's CD-ROM and can be printed and photocopied. These measures can serve as prompts for the clinician but are *not* required for the delivery of the session. Beliefs endorsed on the measures can be directly applied within the session. The clinician can decide whether to focus on the questionnaire responses or to elicit individual beliefs out loud during the session.

Responses on the measures can be reviewed pre- and post-intervention in order to assess whether the client's beliefs were modified as a result of participating in the intervention session. For program directors or clinicians seeking outcomes, these measures can be excellent tools for evaluating this protocol and how effectively clinicians are delivering it.

Often, it's advisable for clients to fill out the questionnaire in advance. It can be mailed to them, or it can be administered by phone. If the client fills it out during the intervention session itself, extra time should be allowed for it.

Development of the Intervention

This evidence-based protocol was originally developed as a tool to increase treatment seeking among individuals with depression in primary care settings. It has since been studied among individuals with depression, post-traumatic stress disorder, and alcohol use disorders.

The protocol was modeled from the theory of planned behavior (TPB) and cognitive theory. TPB postulates that any behavior (in this case, scheduling a mental health or addiction treatment session) depends on three types of beliefs. They are (1) *behavioral beliefs* about the likely consequences of the behavior; (2) *normative beliefs* about the normative expectations of others; and (3) *control beliefs* about the factors that facilitate or prevent the behavior (Ajzen 1991). According to the theory, in brief, behavioral beliefs produce an attitude toward the behavior. Normative beliefs combine to produce perceived social pressure to perform the behavior. Control beliefs affect one's perceived ability to perform the behavior. These three combine to form a general intention of performing the behavior. According to TPB, people who *intend* to engage in a particular behavior, such as entering treatment for a mental health or substance use disorder, are more likely to actually engage in that behavior. The model is illustrated in the figure on the next page.

The theory of planned behavior is complex, and it is recommended that clinicians read further about it to familiarize themselves with its structure and stages. Aside from reading the author's book and selected papers, the clinician can also find additional information about the TPB diagram shown here on the web page "Icek Ajzen: Theory of Planned Behavior" at www.people.umass.edu/aizen/tpb.html.

People who *intend* to engage in a particular behavior, such as entering treatment for a mental health or substance use disorder, are more likely to actually do so.

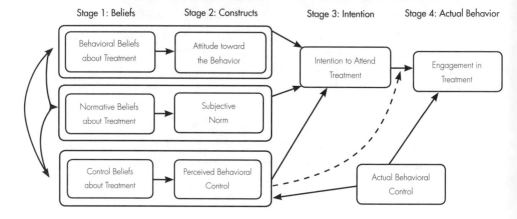

The four stages in the figure can briefly be described as follows:

Stage 1: *Beliefs* could represent the advantages and disadvantages of going to treatment.	**Stage 2:** *Constructs* means the overall or sum of beliefs or attitudes about treatment.
Stage 3: *Intention* represents the idea of whether one wants to attend treatment.	**Stage 4:** *Actual behavior* represents what the client will do or decide about treatment.

In our study for this intervention, we found TPB useful for identifying beliefs about mental health and specialty addiction treatment. In order to actually change behavior, we implemented cognitive theory, which focuses on modifying beliefs in order to modify behavior. Both of these theories postulate that *underlying beliefs predict behavior.* Therefore, one can reason that modifying underlying beliefs would potentially modify behavior. In terms of mental health and addiction treatment, underlying beliefs would also predict treatment-seeking behavior.

For example, an individual resistant to alcohol treatment may state:

1. I do not have a severe drinking problem and do not need treatment.

2. None of my friends have been to alcohol treatment.

3. I don't know if my insurance would cover alcohol treatment, and I don't have any money.

Underlying
beliefs predict
behavior.

According to the above theory, these beliefs lead to a low intention of seeking alcohol treatment. However, these beliefs can be modified in an intervention session to enable the client to increase his or her intention of seeking treatment.

Other Points to Remember

There are four important concerns for the clinician administering the single-session intervention.

Beliefs can be
modified in an
intervention
session to
enable the
individual to
increase his or
her intention
of seeking
treatment.

1. *Elicit active participation.* It is important for the client to be actively involved in the intervention session. Active participation must be requested throughout the entire session by the clinician.

15

2. *Suggest therapy as appropriate.* If the client brings up relevant therapeutic information, ask him or her to consider discussing these symptoms with a trained therapist. Offer the reminder that therapy is a safe place to discuss these issues, while the purpose of today's session is to discuss meeting with a mental health or addiction specialist.

3. *Acknowledge ambivalence.* If the client becomes disengaged during the session, or somehow seems resistant to discussing his or her beliefs, be willing to discuss this ambivalence with the client. Ambivalence could become the focus of the intervention at any time during the session.

4. *Emphasize the positive.* Any positive affirmation should be emphasized. Reinforce any positive self-statement by asking the person to repeat it; then repeat what you heard being said yourself.

The next three parts of this manual encompass the three parts of the intervention session itself (see the chart on page 11 suggesting how the time be spent during the session). Each part has specific goals, timing, and in some cases handouts. Over time, once the clinician becomes more comfortable and experienced in administering this intervention, whether on the phone or in person, he or she will grow less dependent on the manual itself. Meanwhile, the clinician shouldn't hesitate to use the manual directly during the session, for example, reading out loud the scenarios and case studies found in the next section.

Intervention Session Outline

Part 1:
The Cognitive-Behavioral Therapy Model

Goal: The purpose of part 1 of the single-session intervention is to present a five- to ten-minute description of cognitive-behavioral therapy. Part 1 is composed of four steps.

Step 1: Introduce Cognitive-Behavioral Therapy (CBT)

To introduce the basic tenet of interconnectivity of thoughts, feelings, and behavior in cognitive-behavioral theory, begin by simply stating to the client:

> **I am going to briefly explain to you some concepts behind the work we will be doing today. This work is based on what is called cognitive-behavioral therapy, or CBT, which is based on the idea that all of our thoughts, feelings, and behaviors are connected. In other words, what you think will affect what you feel and how you act or behave.**

Step 2: Introduce Handout 1, "Thoughts— Feelings—Behaviors"

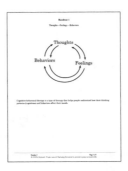

Give the client handout 1. (All handouts can be found on the CD-ROM accompanying this manual. They can be printed and photocopied for your use.) Begin by saying that the illustration on the handout simply helps us visualize and understand the cognitive behavioral process. As you point to the arrows, explain how a thought leads to a feeling (outer circle) and then to a behavior, and how in turn that behavior can then lead to another feeling (inner circle) and thought. It's best to provide examples (see step 3) to illustrate the interconnectedness of thoughts, feelings, and behaviors as construed in cognitive-behavioral therapy.

Step 3: Provide Examples to the Client

Examples always facilitate learning. So present an example of the relationship between thoughts, feelings, and behaviors as illustrated in the previous step. For instance, say:

I'm going to give you an example of how our thoughts influence and lead to feelings and behaviors. Let's consider the illustration I just showed you. Imagine that there are three people—persons A, B, and C—who look at the illustration. Here's what each of them says:

Person A: "Wow! This diagram makes sense. I think I understand how this thought and feeling stuff works" *(thought)*.
Person A feels excited and says, "I'm enjoying learning about this!" *(feeling)* and decides to actively participate in the session *(behavior)*.

Person B: "Okay. The diagram sort of makes sense, but I really don't know what this is all about" *(thought)*.
Person B says he feels doubtful *(feeling)* and decides to sit back and absorb more of the session before becoming active *(behavior)*.

Person C: "This diagram and stuff is all psycho mumbo jumbo" *(thought)*.
Person C says he feels "a bit annoyed" about it all *(feeling)* and decides to disconnect from the discussion and remains silent *(behavior)*.

Step 4: Discuss the Examples

At this point, the client should intuitively sense some difference between the three reactions in the thoughts, feelings, and behaviors of persons A, B, and C. Begin a discussion, feeling free to use the following script:

> As you can see, these three people—A, B, and C—had three different behaviors based on their initial beliefs about the diagram. Person A believed that the diagram made sense and became more involved in the session. Person B believed that more was going to come and decided to wait before becoming more active in the session. Person C believed that the diagram was psychological nonsense and decided to become passive or disengaged from the session. Do you see how this happens with each person? Does this example help you understand better how our different thoughts influence how we feel and behave?

Give the client a chance to respond. It may be helpful to provide another example, such as this one:

> Here's another example that illustrates the relationship between thoughts, feelings, and behavior. Consider what you think and believe when you are sick with a cold. Do you think, "I'm always sick" or "I can never feel good"? What do you do when you think these negative thoughts? Do you do anything to try to feel better? Do you go back to bed,

thinking, "Why bother?" or "What difference does it make—I might as well go to work"? How would these behaviors make you feel?

Is there another way to think about having a cold? What if you instead thought, "I'll go to bed early tonight and get a good night's rest—maybe I'll feel better in the morning," or "I must have caught a cold from a colleague at work who was sick—I need to do better self-care and hygiene at work," or "Oh well, it happens to everyone—I'll take some medicine, lie low, and get some rest." Do you see how different these thoughts are, and how more positive feelings and behaviors can result?

If the client seems to understand the basic relationship between thoughts, feelings, and behaviors, move on to the next section.

Part 2:

The Relationship between Beliefs and Behavior

Goal: The purpose of part 2 is to briefly give more information to underscore the ways thoughts connect with feelings and behaviors. This connection, illustrated in handout 1, is critical to guiding decision making, so the clinician should spend additional time to help anchor the client's understanding of CBT. Part 2 is composed of three steps. Steps 2 and 3 are optional; use them if the client needs more explanation of the interconnectivity of thoughts, feelings, and behaviors, and the constructive or destructive effects of beliefs.

Step 1: Introduce Handout 2, "Constructive and Destructive Thoughts"

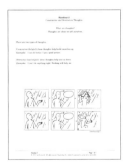

Give the client handout 2, an illustration of a person in the rain. Explain that the illustration is a pictorial example of the way varying thoughts can impact us. This illustration should be used to explain the two types of thoughts, constructive and destructive ones. Use the following script with your client to illustrate how beliefs can impact a person:

Thoughts are ideas that we tell ourselves. In general, there are two types of thoughts. Constructive or positive thoughts are those that help build ourselves up, such as "I can do something to help myself." On the other hand, destructive or negative thoughts tend to tear us down, such as "Nothing will help me." Look at this illustration of a person caught in the rain. Can you tell that the person seems to have two options for thinking about the rain? One thought is destructive, and the other is constructive. Well, we are here today to help you think about different ways to view mental health or addiction treatment, just as the person in the illustration thinks about rain in different ways.

Step 2: Introduce Handout 3, "Eleven Types of Destructive Thoughts" (optional)

Introduce handout 3 with the following script:

> In this handout, you will see a list of eleven types of destructive thoughts. I am giving you this handout for you to read later, if you are interested. We will only briefly review it today. However, I would like for you to have this additional information about how our thinking habits can get us into trouble. It may come in handy for you later.

Step 3: Briefly Review the Types of Destructive Thoughts (optional)

To begin your brief introduction of the destructive thoughts, say to the client:

> In this handout 3, there is a diagram that lists eleven common types of destructive thoughts. These can lead to problematic behaviors, such as avoiding treatment. These thoughts include:

1. All or nothing thinking: We believe something is either completely good or completely bad.

2. Negative filter: We focus only on the negative aspects of a situation.

3. Pessimism: We believe that nothing positive will ever happen.

4. **Exaggerating:** We overemphasize a particular aspect of a situation.

5. **Overgeneralization:** We link related phenomena instead of viewing individual aspects of each phenomenon. We jump to conclusions about related facts or situations without looking at them carefully.

6. **Labeling:** We attach a negative label to something, despite its positive aspects.

7. **Blaming oneself:** We fault ourselves for all problems.

8. **Not giving oneself credit:** We fail to acknowledge ourselves for positive things.

9. **Mind reading:** We believe we understand what someone else is thinking about us without checking the facts.

10. **Negative fortune telling:** We believe we can predict the future, and bad things will happen.

11. **"Shoulding" ourself:** We attach an unrealistic expectation to a situation.

Part 3:

Alternative Ways to Think

Goal: The purpose of part 3 is to coach clients in generating alternative beliefs to replace their existing ones—the ones that keep them from considering change or treatment. Part 3 is composed of eight steps.

Cognitive-behavioral therapy emphasizes that beliefs are modifiable. Some beliefs are fairly open to modification, and it is easy to generate alternatives. For example, it is easy to generate alternative beliefs to the statement "Everyone should always love me." Some beliefs are more resistant to change, and it can be difficult to imagine alternative ways to think, for example, the belief "I wish I didn't have that experience." A person might find that belief to be 100 percent true, and difficult to alter.

This final part of the intervention contains the core practice for guiding decision making among clients. It may be helpful to have the client complete the PASS questionnaire *before* beginning this intervention, either in person or on the phone. It can also be mailed to the client before the intervention, or the client can fill out the questionnaire as part of the one-hour session, though additional time should then be allowed.

Step 1: Introduce Handout 4A, "Worksheet: Alternative Ways to Think"

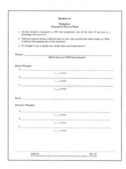

Give handout 4A to the client and introduce it as a worksheet that will be used in the remaining time of the session. Review the three numbered points at the top of the handout with the client, stating how they are essential to changing one's thoughts.

CLINICAL NOTE: As noted above, part 3 contains the core information for addressing negative or destructive beliefs, and creating new and more helpful ones. Before the session, it may be wise to review "Solutions for Potential Problems That May Arise during the Intervention Session" and "Case Examples" (appendices A and B). Until the clinician has developed more familiarity and expertise with this intervention, it is recommended these two items be reviewed before each new client.

Step 2: Provide Examples of How Thoughts Affect Feelings

Give the client an example of how thoughts and beliefs lead to certain feelings, and how a person might then modify his or her beliefs to change those feelings. You may use the following script:

> **In cognitive behavioral-therapy, therapists help people change the way they behave. They also help people change what they think, so that they are less depressed or anxious. Handout 4A is a worksheet called "Alternative Ways to Think." With this worksheet, we can analyze how we respond to events in our lives. First, let's use it to see how particular events provoke certain feelings, thoughts, or behaviors.**
>
> **Here's a simple example: You're driving down the highway and a police siren turns on right behind you. The siren is the event. Your first thought might be, "Uh-oh. I'm speeding."** (On the handout, point to the heading "Thought.") **What are the results of that thought? A result might be a feeling, like anxiety.** (Point to the heading "Result.") **A result might also be a behavior, such as slowing down your speed.**
>
> **Here's another possible response to the same situation. Your first thought might be, "That jerk better not pull me over. He should be out catching real criminals rather than sitting here trying to give me a speeding ticket."** (Point to the "Thought" heading again.)

The feeling that results from that thought would be anger. (Point to the "Result" heading.) Another result might be a behavior: you pound your fists against the steering wheel. If the police car pulls you over for speeding, you might direct your anger at the highway patrolman for doing his job—and that's not usually the best way to get out of a speeding ticket.

Now, let's say the police officer drives by without stopping you. What are you feeling now? Still angry? Not likely. You probably feel relieved, maybe even elated. You think, "I'm off the hook!" and your feelings change in an instant. This is an example of how your thoughts affect your feelings, which can in turn affect your behavior.

Step 3: Review Handout 4B, "Sample Worksheet 1: Alternative Ways to Think"

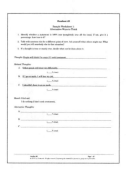

Using this sample worksheet, the client may be able to better understand how to complete his or her own handout 4A with the clinician's help. To begin, give the client a copy of handout 4B and explain that this version of the worksheet has been filled out to show an imaginary person's situation. Now, ask the client to imagine a person who is considering getting treatment for a mental health problem. Ask the client to be specific and say what gender and age this person is. Then, introduce the following sample:

> **Okay. Let's imagine this person being reluctant about seeking treatment. Let's imagine what he might be thinking about it. He might think, "People will think I'm crazy if I seek treatment." So, in this sample, you see that thought listed next to the heading "Thought."** (Point to that heading on handout 4B.)

Thought: People will think I'm crazy if I seek treatment.

Then, without directing the client's attention to the next lines on the handout, ask:

> **What other thoughts might come to this person's mind along with the idea of being seen as crazy? What does that thought mean to you? What is the worst thing that could happen if people saw you as crazy for**

getting treatment? Let's both consider three other related thoughts that our imaginary person might have.

Brainstorm with the client until you have at least three additional related thoughts.

> **CLINICAL NOTE:** You need not write these brainstormed thoughts down, since three "related thoughts" already appear on the handout.

Say to the client:

Okay, in our sample worksheet you can see three related thoughts the person might have. These thoughts appear in the appropriate blanks under the heading "Related Thoughts." (Point to that section on the handout.)

Related Thoughts:

A. Other people will treat me differently.

B. If I go on meds, I will lose my job.

C. I shouldn't have to go on meds.

Now, ask the client:

How do you feel, or how might the imaginary person feel, when I read these thoughts out loud? These feelings appear under

the heading "Result," because the feeling resulted from the thought. (Point to that line in the handout.)

Result: I feel sad.

Write down the feelings mentioned by the client. Remind the client that results can be behaviors as well as feelings. Ask:

What kind of behavior occurs as a result of having these thoughts and feelings? (Point to the *Result* line.)

Result: I do nothing (I don't seek treatment).

Step 4: Fill Out Handout 4A, "Worksheet: Alternative Ways to Think"

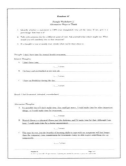

In this step, tell the client that he or she is ready to fill out his or her own worksheet and to record thoughts, feelings, and behaviors. Use handout

4A, which was discussed earlier. Use the client's PASS questionnaire, section 2, to identify some negative thoughts (beliefs) that the person holds. Select one and have the person record it under the heading "Thought." If the client did not fill out the PASS scale, have the person identify his or her own thought's about treatment for mental health or substance use. Use the following script to guide the person:

> **Here is what we will do with this handout. We've already practiced once, asking ourselves how an imaginary person might think, feel, and behave. Now, let's fill out the form for real, for yourself. We are going to select a thought from the PASS questionnaire you just filled out (on the phone or in person), and we are going to apply it to this model.**

Next to the heading "Thought," have the person write down a thought (belief) chosen from the questionnaire (or one elicited from the discussion). Or the clinician can do the writing.

To elicit "related thoughts," ask the client to describe other thoughts that he or she has about the thought, as done in the previous sample exercise. (See Step 6 for tips on eliciting related and alternative thoughts.) Have the person record three related thoughts in the appropriate location on the form.

Step 5: Score the Accuracy of Related Thoughts to Identify Alternative Thoughts

The next part of the assignment is to determine alternatives to a client's specific "automatic thoughts" about seeking treatment. To start this process, first ask the client to gauge the accuracy of each related thought listed on the form:

I want you to do three things with your related thoughts. First, I first want you to tell me whether each thought is absolutely 100 percent true, 100 percent of the time. Are there any facts that contradict the thought? Second, I want you to think about whether other people would share this same type of thought. What would you tell somebody else in that situation? And third, if that thought is mostly true, I want you to think about what can be done about it.

Let's look at each related thought and decide how true it is. Let's start with the first one. How much of the time is this a true and accurate thought? If it is not true 100 percent of the time, what is true for the rest of the time? What other thoughts are true? If the thought isn't entirely true, but only true half of the time, what is true the other half of the time? Is there evidence that does *not* support this thought? Do you know of someone who would not support

**this thought? What would that person think
is true?**

As the client identifies the percentage for each
thought, write it down on the handout.

Step 6: Determine Alternative Thoughts

This step is the *most critical step* of the intervention session. It is at this point that the client will
further consider seeking treatment. It is important to process through each related thought and
either determine alternative thoughts for each, or
problem solve. A particular thought might be completely true; however, additional information may
balance out that thought so that it does not impact
behavior—so think creatively to help "unstick" any
problematic thoughts.

The most effective way to help clients identify
alternative thoughts is to ask them to reconsider
and restate their related thoughts. If the thought
is not 100 percent true (for example, "Everyone will
think I am crazy for seeking treatment"), then ask
the client to reframe it in a way that would be 100
percent true (for example, "Well, my spouse wants
me to get some help, but my friend Harry doesn't").

Another method of generating alternative thoughts
is to offer the client contradictory facts. If a client
states a thought that is not supported by information
their peers had given on the questionnaire, tell
the client about it. For example, if a client says,
"Everyone in the military would think I was crazy

for seeking treatment," they can be given the information that a high percentage of their peers in the military reported that they would not perceive themselves as crazy for seeking treatment. The clinician can provide other pertinent information if the client is non-military or civilian.

You could also use the following questions to help clients generate alternative thoughts. Adapted from Christine Padesky and Dennis Greenberger's *Clinician's Guide to Mind Over Mood*, these questions can be used to find evidence that does not support clients' related thoughts.

1. Are there experiences that show this thought is not completely true all the time?
2. If my best friend or someone I love had this thought, what would I tell them?
3. If my best friend or someone who loves me knew I was thinking this thought, what would they say to me? What evidence would they point out to me that would suggest that my thoughts were not 100 percent true?
4. When I am not feeling this way, do I think about this type of situation any differently? How?
5. When I have felt this way in the past, what did I think about that helped me feel better?
6. Have I been in this type of situation before? What happened? Is there anything different between this situation and previous ones? What have I learned from prior experiences that could help me now?

7. Are there any small things that contradict my thoughts that I might be discounting as not important?

8. Five years from now, if I look back on this situation, will I look at it any differently? Will I focus on any different part of my experience?

9. Are there any strengths or positives about this situation that I am ignoring?

10. Am I jumping to conclusions that are not completely justified by the evidence?

11. Am I blaming myself for something over which I do not have complete control?

Once a list of alternative thoughts has been established, ask the client:

How do you feel when I read these thoughts out loud?

Write down the *feelings* the client states. Then ask:

What kinds of behavior occur as a result of having these thoughts and feelings?

Write down the *behaviors* the client states.

This process should be completed for a maximum of four different thoughts. It is important to reinforce any positive statement the client makes. Repeat any such statement back to the client, so he or she understands that you heard it and has time to recognize its value.

Step 7: Review Handout 4C, "Sample Worksheet 2: Alternative Ways to Think"

Give handout 4C, "Sample Worksheet 2: Alternative

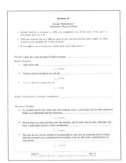

Ways to Think" to the client so he or she can view a complete example of developing alternative beliefs about mental health treatment. Review this handout with the client.

Step 8: Conclusion

In concluding the session, affirm the client's decisions to change his or her behaviors. First summarize what the person has learned in this intervention about thoughts and beliefs and their connection to feelings and behaviors. Depending on what new thoughts the person has developed about mental health or substance abuse treatment, you might say:

Okay, it sounds like you are more interested in seeking treatment now than you were in the beginning of this session. Do you know how you can contact a person to help you with your next step? Do you know whom to call in your area? You can make that phone call now, if you'd like, or later when you're home. If you need any additional help or discussion, I'm here. Is there anything else standing in the way of your making that call?

If the person needs a referral, make one. If he or she feels confident enough to take the next step, then congratulate the person and conclude your session.

Appendix A:

Solutions for Potential Problems That May Arise during the Intervention Session

In these five common situations, many clinicians have found that these guidelines help them keep the session productive.

1. *Client is emotionally vulnerable.* The process of modifying beliefs about initiating mental health and/or addiction treatment is provocative. Often, clients express vulnerability toward the end of the intervention session. This feeling may be both unexpected and uncomfortable for them. For the clinician, it's important to acknowledge this emotional vulnerability. It may be a healthy sign that the client is ready for mental health or addiction treatment services to begin, and is emotionally open to the process for the first time. While some clients may feel excited to experience their feelings about entering treatment, others feel fear. For those experiencing fear, it is important to let the person discuss this fear during the session. Clinicians should also suggest that they discuss any such difficulties with their future therapist.

   While some clients may feel excited to experience their feelings about entering treatment, others feel fear.

2. *Client claims to be fully ready to seek treatment.* Some clients will begin the intervention session stating that they are completely open to treatment

and have decided to go. It is important to acknowledge this decision and still proceed with the intervention session. Some clients express positive beliefs about mental health or addiction treatment. Typically, clients presenting in this way have decided to go to treatment, yet there is still one aspect of their disorder holding them back. Clinicians should help such clients process completely through their beliefs about treatment, so that they actually make an appointment for treatment instead of only saying they will do so.

> It is important to acknowledge a decision to enter treatment and still proceed with the intervention session.

3. *Client strongly resists seeking treatment.* On the other hand, some clients clearly indicate during the session that they will not seek treatment. This is also important to acknowledge. In this case, ask what would have to happen to prompt them to seek treatment. Answering this question, clients often describe certain consequences of their substance use or symptoms. For example, clients might say that they would only consider seeking treatment if they lost their job or got a DUI. These consequences can be disastrous. It's important for these clients to understand that they're choosing to risk the consequences, rather than working to avoid the consequences altogether. Other people resist because they believe that problems should be handled privately, and seeking help is a sign of weakness. The same dialogue can be helpful here. Handling it alone might be the preferred option, yet at the risk of what consequence? This discussion does not have

> It's important for these clients to understand that they're choosing to risk the consequences, rather than working to avoid the consequences altogether.

to be confrontational, yet it is important to probe for the specifics of their plan down the road. If treatment is not an option until they experience the consequence that they dread, discuss with them what they might do if the consequence happens two years from now. What would they do at that point? What would their beliefs about treatment be then?

4. *Client has difficulty generating alternative beliefs.* In this case, it is acceptable for the clinician to offer prompts for generating these beliefs. Ultimately, however, it is best for clients to modify their own beliefs as much as possible.

5. *Client has modest goals.* Many clients initiate treatment with the goal of eliminating distress and suffering, but some resist treatment because they claim to prefer suffering with the disorder. This is most frequently seen in those suffering from substance use disorders. Often clients express a desire to lessen the impact of their disorder, rather than be completely free of it. Ultimately, it is important to acknowledge the client's goal for seeking treatment.

Appendix B:
Case Examples

These case studies illustrate how three clients grew in self-awareness during the intervention. Together with a clinician, all three filled out the "Alternative Ways to Think" worksheets which are included here. (Names and identifying details have been changed.)

John

John is a twenty-seven-year-old who served in the war in Iraq with the Army National Guard. John has been involved with the National Guard for the past seven years and joined the military to serve his country in national emergencies such as natural disasters; he also hopes to use college tuition benefits. John was not opposed to serving during a time of war; however, he has a wife and two young children. During his year-long deployment in Iraq, John served as a bomb hunter. He had several traumatic experiences there, including surviving an explosion that killed several Iraqis—women and children among them—and finding an improvised explosive device that failed to explode. He recounts these episodes in detail, yet reports very little anxiety over them. In fact, his only main complaint is that he can't stop replaying the episodes in his mind.

John screened positive for PTSD and alcohol abuse, but denies the need for treatment because he is "not experiencing any anxiety." Instead, he reports feeling numb and unemotional. He is having difficulty in relationships and is not performing well on his job because he "doesn't care" about it. Because he has no anxiety over his symptoms, treatment would be pointless, he said. When John was asked to identify his beliefs about engaging in treatment for his intrusive memories, he said he had three related thoughts. First, even though the picture of the trauma was going constantly through his mind, the picture wasn't bothering him. Second, going to treatment would mean that he was weak. And third, treatment couldn't help him deal with anger or anxiety, because he wasn't having any.

During the intervention, John was asked to elaborate on each of these thoughts more deliberately. For example, his first thought—the constant replaying of the trauma—seemed problematic even if he couldn't identify or feel his anxiety about it. The clinician probed, wondering whether the recurring thoughts interfered with his ability to concentrate at work or at home. John admitted that there were situations at home that felt stupid, considering what he had been through. One example was his ability to prepare dinner for his wife. Before he was deployed, John liked to cook dinner for his wife; he also liked leaving her notes expressing his love for her. But he doesn't prepare meals anymore, John said. He has to make sure all the doors are locked and his weapons are loaded, instead of wasting time cooking dinner. His wife is upset by the difference, and she doesn't understand the change in his behavior. But even though she is upset, John claims he lacks enough emotion to engage in those meaningless activities. Next, John and the clinician explored the idea that the activities he now engages in are an expression of love. Since safety seemed to be a core issue for him post-deployment, perhaps his checking doors and weapons could be construed as an expression of love for his family. Further, it could be understood in emotional terms: he was expressing his love and concern over the safety of himself and his family. He was able to agree with this assessment and restated his first thought as, "I am having recurring thoughts about the trauma, which interfere with my ability to communicate well with my family."

John's second thought was that going to treatment would mean that he was weak. Since treatment means that you have to talk with another individual about your problems, that made it a weakness in John's eyes. It's better to not have others know what you struggle with, he said, so they can't use it against you in the future. John admitted that he got this idea from his father, who never complained about his problems. John also admitted that his father's problems were never resolved and probably could have been. With this assessment, John restated that he still believes that "going to therapy means that you are weak, but it could also mean that you are trying to take care of your issues."
John's third thought—about the absence of anger and anxiety—was reframed during the discussion

of the first thought. John was able to admit having anxiety but said that he pushes it away to focus on other things (such as the recurring memories of the trauma). He still struggles with his perception of anxiety and how it is expressed, but he was able to see that his expression of anxiety and anger may be different from what he thought. He reframed his third thought this way: "I am having some anxiety, but it is hard to feel it because I am preoccupied with my thoughts about Iraq."

When John was asked to look at his three new thoughts and talk further about the decision to engage in treatment, he admitted that he might benefit from talking to someone. He said that he was not happy with the state of his marriage and wanted things to get better, but didn't know how to work on it. He also stated that he wanted to be able to stop his thoughts from preoccupying so much of his time.

John's worksheet can be found on the next page.

John's Worksheet

Thought: I don't need treatment.

Related Thoughts:

A. The trauma isn't causing me anxiety. (75% true)

B. Going to treatment means that I am weak. (95% true)

C. Treatment can't help with the anxiety or anger because I'm not feeling any. (70% true)

Result: I feel numb.

Alternative Thoughts:

A. I am having recurring thoughts about the trauma, which interfere with my ability to communicate well with my family. (100% true)

B. I still believe that going to therapy means that you are weak, but it could also mean that you are trying to take care of your issues. (100% true)

C. I am having some anxiety, but it is hard to feel it because I am preoccupied with my thoughts about Iraq. (100% true)

Steve

A musician who plays in a band, Steve is a twenty-two-year-old male who screened positive for alcohol dependence. During the intervention session, Steve stated that he is not considering seeking treatment but does believe he has a drinking problem. He has experienced several consequences from his alcohol use, including broken bones, a DUI violation, and losing friends. But, said Steve, alcohol treatment is not an option for him at this time: "Alcohol treatment is for people who have serious alcohol problems." His automatic thought about treatment was that he could handle his problem on his own. When asked what he believed would help him with his drinking, he stated: (1) "I can control my drinking on my own," (2) "I have a support group [of family and friends] that is helping me," and (3) "My alcohol problem is really only a problem when I drink hard liquor."

When asked to elaborate on his belief that he could control his drinking on his own, Steve indicated that when he tours with his band, he is able to control his alcohol intake; he only drinks when he is around others who are partying. Throughout the discussion, Steve was able to see that his drinking occurs when he puts himself in certain situations (such as parties with alcohol present). In those contexts, he said, he has absolutely no ability to say no and will drink heavily. In other contexts, such as with his band mates, he can abstain. Steve modified his initial belief from "I can control my drinking on my own" to "I can only control my drinking if I am in a certain environment. I often choose to go to parties where I can drink, because parties and drinking are more fun. At parties, I cannot control my drinking."

In terms of his second belief regarding his support group of family and friends, Steve admitted that he often has blackouts and memory loss. In those cases, Steve said, he appreciates it when his dad and others tell him that they are disappointed in his behavior. He believes it helps when his friends tell him what he did, so he can see how bad he was. When asked what happens when his friends say they didn't like how he acted, Steve replied that he often lies in return, telling them that he has recently quit or cut back. This fact suggests that even though he believes his family and friends are helping him by disapproving, their statements are actually not very effective at changing the behavior. Steve modified his second belief to "My support group is supportive of me but not very effective at helping me change my drinking habits."

Steve's third belief was that he blacks out and has negative consequences from drinking only when he drinks hard liquor. Steve was easily able to modify this belief by amending it to "Liquor isn't the only problem. I've gotten really sick from drinking lots of beer."

At this point in the intervention, Steve said he didn't really understand what options were available to treat alcohol use disorders. He knew about inpatient treatment and Alcoholics Anonymous (AA) but was unfamiliar with other options. Other options such as individual therapy and outpatient treatment were discussed. Steve began to investigate the idea of individual therapy so that he can discuss some of his struggles with a professional, maintaining his belief that he is handling his problem on his own.

Steve's worksheet can be found on the next page.

Steve's Worksheet

Thought: I can handle the problem on my own, so I don't need treatment.

Related Thoughts:

    A. I can control my drinking on my own. (25% true)

    B. I have a support group that is helping me. (50% true)

    C. My alcohol problem is really only a problem when I drink hard liquor. (0% true)

Result: I feel optimistic.

Alternative Thoughts:

    A. I can only control my drinking if I am in a certain environment. I often choose to go to parties where I can drink, because parties and drinking are more fun. At parties, I cannot control my drinking. (100% true)

    B. My support group is supportive of me but not very effective at helping me change my drinking habits. (100% true)

    C. Liquor isn't the only problem. I've gotten really sick from drinking lots of beer. (100% true)

Kimberly

A thirty-nine-year-old physician with alcohol dependence disorder, Kimberly is very resistant to seeking treatment. Because she is a physician, she believes that she has a thorough understanding of addiction and should be able to control the problem on her own. Kimberly has two young children and is married, but spends most of her time working. When she is not at work, she consumes large quantities of alcohol in order to sleep. She believes that she is a "functional alcoholic" and that no one who knows her would believe that she has a drinking problem. She claims that she is never impaired despite the amount she drinks. She has a family history of alcoholism: everyone in her family drank, and no one quit or sought help. In fact, when Kimberly was twelve, her father died from an alcohol-related injury. People in her family would be surprised at how much she drinks, she said, because she is so functional.

Kimberly participated in the intervention session at her husband's request. She wants to show him that she is willing to discuss treatment so he'll stop harassing her about it. She reports that her children both say that they want her to stop drinking, but that she is a good mom because she reads them a story each night before bedtime.

Kimberly indicated that her automatic thought about treatment is that going to treatment would ruin her career. Her patients and colleagues would think less of her, she said, if she admitted that she had a problem with alcohol. She believes that she should be able to quit on her own and that she already knows everything that would be discussed in a treatment session.

In a discussion of her belief that treatment would ruin her career, it became apparent that Kimberly has had some difficulty at work as a result of her drinking. Because she has trouble remembering patient-related issues, she tries to record patient information in great detail immediately after each visit. This has led to problems being on time for subsequent patient visits, which gets her into trouble with administrative personnel. After an extensive discussion about her inability to separate work from her drinking, she modified her belief this way: "My professional career may be in jeopardy as a result of my drinking, and I would like to do what I can to save it, although I would prefer that no one from work ever knows that I have this problem." Additionally, she identified several physicians she respects and admires who are open about being in recovery from addiction, and she admits that their careers were not damaged as a result of seeking treatment.

The idea that seeking treatment is a sign of weakness is often reported, especially among professionals and men in the military. Kimberly modified her belief about weakness as, "I am acting more like a patient in need of treatment than the professional that I am." Related to this belief was the idea that since she is already educated about addiction, she would not benefit from these services. This belief was modified to "Although I will probably know everything academic about addiction, I seem to have difficulty applying it to my own behavior and may have a little to learn."

Kimberly determined that the decision to seek help was potentially disastrous to her career, although it was better than staying on her current course, which had the potential to ruin her family, health, and career anyway.

Kimberly's worksheet can be found on the next page.

Kimberly's Worksheet

Thought: Going to treatment will ruin my career.

Related Thoughts:

A. My patients and colleagues will think less of me if I admit I have a problem with alcohol. (85% true)

B. I should be able to quit on my own. (90% true)

C. Professionally, I know about addiction. (100% true)

Result: I feel frustrated.

Alternative Thoughts:

A. My professional career may be in jeopardy as a result of my drinking, and I would like to do what I can to save it, although I would prefer that no one from work ever knows that I have this problem. (100% true)

B. I am acting more like a patient in need of treatment than the professional that I am. (100% true)

C. Although I will probably know everything academic about addiction, I seem to have difficulty applying it to my own behavior and may have a little to learn. (90% true)

Appendix C:

Perceptions about Services Scale
(PASS Questionnaire)

Description: What are your general impressions of mental health treatment, and what does that mean for you? This questionnaire helps you consider those topics. At some time in their lives, many people seek help for concerns such as depression, anxiety, substance use concerns, and post-traumatic stress disorder (PTSD). In this questionnaire, the term "mental health treatment" could refer to simply visiting a primary care doctor or a mental health specialist to discuss such concerns. This questionnaire is voluntary and confidential. Only the clinician will see your responses.

Instructions: Please read and answer each question. Section 1 asks for basic information about you. Section 2 asks about your thoughts on the possibility of seeking mental health treatment.

ID # _____ Date: _____
Interviewer Initials: _____

Section 1

1. Are you

    ❑ Female
    ❑ Male

2. What is your age? _____

    ❑ Don't know
    ❑ Refuse to answer

3. What is your race?

   ❏ African American
   ❏ Asian American
   ❏ Caucasian
   ❏ Native American
   ❏ Other _____
   ❏ Don't know
   ❏ Refuse to answer

4. Do you consider yourself of Hispanic or Latino/a descent?

   ❏ Yes
   ❏ No
   ❏ Don't know
   ❏ Refuse to answer

5. What type of health care insurance do you currently use?

   ❏ Tricare / Tricare for Life
   ❏ Medicaid
   ❏ Medicare
   ❏ Private
   ❏ Other _____
   ❏ Uninsured
   ❏ Don't know
   ❏ Refuse to answer

6. From your home, about how long does it take to get to your primary care doctor?

   ❏ 0 to 30 minutes
   ❏ 31 to 60 minutes
   ❏ More than 61 minutes
   ❏ No doctor
   ❏ Don't know
   ❏ Refuse to answer

7. Have you ever seen a health care provider about mental health concerns?

 ❏ Yes
 ❏ No
 ❏ Don't know
 ❏ Refuse to answer

8. If you have recently been in the military, have you seen a health care provider about mental health concerns since your deployment? (Skip this question if it doesn't apply to you.)

 ❏ Yes
 ❏ No
 ❏ Don't know
 ❏ Refuse to answer

9. Are you currently taking any medication for mental health problems?

 ❏ Yes
 ❏ No
 ❏ Don't know
 ❏ Refuse to answer

Section 2

In this section, answer the questions on the scales below: for example, the first scale ranges from "Strongly Disagree" to "Strongly Agree." Fill in the circle that best represents your answer. (Remember, seeking help often starts with a small step. In this questionnaire the term "mental health treatment" could refer to simply visiting a primary care doctor or a mental health specialist to discuss your concerns.)

10. If I went to mental health treatment, I would have fewer bothersome symptoms (I would get better).

Strongly Disagree ○ ○ ○ ○ ○ ○ ○ Strongly Agree

11. If I went to mental health treatment, people would think I was crazy.

Strongly Disagree ○ ○ ○ ○ ○ ○ ○ Strongly Agree

12. Going to mental health treatment would mean that I cannot handle problems on my own.

Strongly Disagree ○ ○ ○ ○ ○ ○ ○ Strongly Agree

13. Going to mental health treatment would hurt my work career.

Strongly Disagree ○ ○ ○ ○ ○ ○ ○ Strongly Agree

14. Going to mental health treatment would hurt my military career.

Strongly Disagree ○ ○ ○ ○ ○ ○ ○ Strongly Agree
(Note: Skip this question if it doesn't apply to you.)

15. Going to mental health treatment would help me identify my triggers and learn to cope better.

Strongly Disagree ○ ○ ○ ○ ○ ○ ○ Strongly Agree
(Note: "Triggers" are the events, places, people, and things that you may react to in an unhealthy way.)

16. For me, identifying my triggers and learning to cope better is

Not Important ○ ○ ○ ○ ○ ○ ○ Extremely Desirable

17. For me, having fewer bothersome symptoms (getting better) is

Not Important ○ ○ ○ ○ ○ ○ ○ Extremely Desirable

18. For me, being able to handle problems on my own is

Not Important ○ ○ ○ ○ ○ ○ ○ Extremely Desirable

19. If people thought I was crazy, this would be

Extremely Undesirable ○ ○ ○ ○ ○ ○ ○ Not Important

20. If my work career were hurt, this would be

Extremely Undesirable ○ ○ ○ ○ ○ ○ ○ Not Important

21. If my military career were hurt, this would be

Extremely Undesirable ○ ○ ○ ○ ○ ○ ○ Not Important
(Note: Skip this question if it doesn't apply to you.)

22. My family would approve of my going to mental health treatment.

Strongly Disagree ○ ○ ○ ○ ○ ○ ○ Strongly Agree

23. People I work with would approve of my going to mental health treatment.

Strongly Disagree ○ ○ ○ ○ ○ ○ ○ Strongly Agree

24. My friends would approve of my going to mental health treatment.

Strongly Disagree ○ ○ ○ ○ ○ ○ ○ Strongly Agree

25. In matters of mental health treatment, the opinions of my family are important to me.

Not at All ○ ○ ○ ○ ○ ○ ○ Very Much

26. In matters of mental health treatment, the opinions of my co-workers are important to me.

Not at All ○ ○ ○ ○ ○ ○ ○ Very Much

27. In matters of mental health treatment, the opinions of my friends are important to me.

Not at All ○ ○ ○ ○ ○ ○ ○ Very Much

28. Some of my experiences would be very difficult to talk about in mental health treatment.

Strongly Disagree ○ ○ ○ ○ ○ ○ ○ Strongly Agree

29. I would be comfortable talking to a mental health specialist.

Strongly Disagree ○ ○ ○ ○ ○ ○ ○ Strongly Agree

30. I could easily get to mental health treatment (transportation is not a problem).

Strongly Disagree ○ ○ ○ ○ ○ ○ ○ Strongly Agree

31. I could make time for going to mental health treatment.

Strongly Disagree ○ ○ ○ ○ ○ ○ ○ Strongly Agree

32. Having difficulty talking about experiences in mental health treatment would make my going to mental health treatment

Easier ○ ○ ○ ○ ○ ○ ○ More Difficult

33. My transportation issues would make going to mental health treatment

    Easier ○ ○ ○ ○ ○ ○ ○ More Difficult

34. My comfort talking to a mental health specialist would make going to mental health treatment

    Easier ○ ○ ○ ○ ○ ○ ○ More Difficult

35. My time issues would make going to mental health treatment

    Easier ○ ○ ○ ○ ○ ○ ○ More Difficult

36. Overall, I think going to mental health treatment for me would be

    a. Worthless ○ ○ ○ ○ ○ ○ ○ Valuable

    b. Harmful ○ ○ ○ ○ ○ ○ ○ Beneficial

    c. Not Therapeutic ○ ○ ○ ○ ○ ○ ○ Therapeutic

    d. Bad ○ ○ ○ ○ ○ ○ ○ Good

37. Most people who are important to me would approve of my going to mental health treatment.

    Definitely True ○ ○ ○ ○ ○ ○ ○ Definitely False

38. It is expected of me that I go to mental health treatment if I need it.

    Definitely True ○ ○ ○ ○ ○ ○ ○ Definitely False

39. People who are close to me would themselves go to mental health treatment if they needed it.

    Definitely True ○ ○ ○ ○ ○ ○ ○ Definitely False

40. For me, going to mental health treatment would be

Possible ○ ○ ○ ○ ○ ○ ○ Impossible

41. If I wanted to, I could easily go to mental health treatment.

Strongly Agree ○ ○ ○ ○ ○ ○ ○ Strongly Disagree

42. Going to mental health treatment is under my control.

Completely ○ ○ ○ ○ ○ ○ ○ Not at All

43. I intend to go to mental health treatment.

Definitely Yes ○ ○ ○ ○ ○ ○ ○ Definitely Not

44. I will try to go to mental health treatment.

Extremely Likely ○ ○ ○ ○ ○ ○ ○ Extremely Unlikely

Appendix D:

Modifying Perceptions about Services Scale
(iMPASS Questionnaire)

Description: What are your general impressions of alcohol treatment, and what does that mean for you? This questionnaire is designed to assess your perceptions of alcohol treatment and use, and will help you consider those topics. Participation is voluntary and confidential. Only the clinician will see your response.

Instructions: Please read and answer each question. **Section 1** asks for basic information about you. **Section 2** asks about your thoughts on the possibility of seeking alcohol treatment.

ID # _____ Date: _____
Interviewer Initials: _____

Section 1

1. Are you
   - ❏ Female
   - ❏ Male

2. What is your age? _____
   - ❏ Don't know
   - ❏ Refuse to answer

3. What is your race?

    ❏ African American
    ❏ Asian American
    ❏ Caucasian
    ❏ Native American
    ❏ Other _____
    ❏ Don't know
    ❏ Refuse to answer

4. Do you consider yourself of Hispanic or Latino/a descent?

    ❏ Yes
    ❏ No
    ❏ Don't know
    ❏ Refuse to answer

5. What type of healthcare insurance do you currently use?

    ❏ Tricare/Tricare for Life
    ❏ Medicaid
    ❏ Medicare
    ❏ Private
    ❏ Other _____
    ❏ Uninsured
    ❏ Don't know
    ❏ Refuse to answer

6. From your home, about how long does it take to get to your primary care doctor?

    ❏ 0 to 30 minutes
    ❏ 31 to 60 minutes
    ❏ More than 61 minutes
    ❏ No doctor
    ❏ Don't know
    ❏ Refuse to answer

7. Are you currently taking any medication for mental health problems?

     ❑ Yes
     ❑ No
     ❑ Don't know
     ❑ Refuse to answer

Section 2

In this section, answer the questions on the scales below: for example, the first scale ranges from "Strongly Disagree" to "Strongly Agree." Fill in the circle that best represents your answer. Alcohol treatment (outpatient, inpatient, AA, group, or private) is a process designed to help individuals deal with an alcohol problem.

8. Going to alcohol treatment would mean that I can't handle problems on my own.

Strongly Disagree ○ ○ ○ ○ ○ ○ ○ Strongly Agree

9. I don't have a problem with alcohol.

Strongly Disagree ○ ○ ○ ○ ○ ○ ○ Strongly Agree

10. I think the problem will go away by itself.

Strongly Disagree ○ ○ ○ ○ ○ ○ ○ Strongly Agree

11. Once my other problems improve (for example, relationship, job, or legal problems), then my drinking problems will go away.

Strongly Disagree ○ ○ ○ ○ ○ ○ ○ Strongly Agree

12. Going to treatment would hurt my work career.

Strongly Disagree ○ ○ ○ ○ ○ ○ ○ Strongly Agree

13. For me, being able to handle problems on my own is

Not Important ○ ○ ○ ○ ○ ○ ○ Extremely Desirable

14. Believing the problem will go away by itself is

Not Important ○ ○ ○ ○ ○ ○ ○ Extremely Desirable

15. Having other problems in my life improve would be

Not Important ○ ○ ○ ○ ○ ○ ○ Extremely Desirable

16. If I thought I had a problem with alcohol, this would be

Extremely Undesirable ○ ○ ○ ○ ○ ○ ○ Not Important

17. If my work career were hurt, this would be

Extremely Undesirable ○ ○ ○ ○ ○ ○ ○ Not Important

18. My family would approve of my going to alcohol treatment.

Strongly Disagree ○ ○ ○ ○ ○ ○ ○ Strongly Agree

19. People I work with would approve of my going to alcohol treatment.

Strongly Disagree ○ ○ ○ ○ ○ ○ ○ Strongly Agree

20. My friends would approve of my going to alcohol treatment.

Strongly Disagree ○ ○ ○ ○ ○ ○ ○ Strongly Agree

21. In matters of alcohol treatment, the opinions of my family are important to me.

    Not at all ○○○○○○○ Very Much

22. In matters of alcohol treatment, the opinions of my co-workers are important to me.

    Not at all ○○○○○○○ Very Much

23. In matters of alcohol treatment, the opinions of my friends are important to me.

    Not at all ○○○○○○○ Very Much

24. Some of my experiences would be very difficult to talk about in alcohol treatment.

    Strongly Disagree ○○○○○○○ Strongly Agree

25. I would be comfortable talking to a alcohol specialist.

    Strongly Disagree ○○○○○○○ Strongly Agree

26. I could afford to go to alcohol treatment.

    Strongly Disagree ○○○○○○○ Strongly Agree

27. I could easily get to alcohol treatment (transportation is not a problem).

    Strongly Disagree ○○○○○○○ Strongly Agree

28. I could make time for going to alcohol treatment.

    Strongly Disagree ○○○○○○○ Strongly Agree

29. Having difficulty talking about experiences in alcohol treatment would make my going to alcohol treatment

    Easier ○○○○○○○ More Difficult

30. Being easily able to get there (no transportation problems) would make me going to alcohol treatment

Easier ○ ○ ○ ○ ○ ○ ○ More Difficult

31. Being comfortable talking to a alcohol specialist would make my going to alcohol treatment

Easier ○ ○ ○ ○ ○ ○ ○ More Difficult

32. Having time available would make my going to alcohol treatment

Easier ○ ○ ○ ○ ○ ○ ○ More Difficult

33. Being able to afford alcohol treatment would make it

Easier ○ ○ ○ ○ ○ ○ ○ More Difficult

34. Overall, I think going to alcohol treatment for me would be

   a.   Worthless ○ ○ ○ ○ ○ ○ ○ Valuable
   b.   Harmful ○ ○ ○ ○ ○ ○ ○ Beneficial
   c.   Not Therapeutic ○ ○ ○ ○ ○ ○ ○ Therapeutic
   d.   Bad ○ ○ ○ ○ ○ ○ ○ Good

35. Most people who are important to me would approve of my going to alcohol treatment.

Definitely True ○ ○ ○ ○ ○ ○ ○ Definitely False

36. It is expected of me that I go to alcohol treatment if I need it.

Definitely True ○ ○ ○ ○ ○ ○ ○ Definitely False

37. People who are close to me would themselves go to alcohol treatment if they needed it.

    Definitely True ○ ○ ○ ○ ○ ○ ○ Definitely False

38. For me, going to alcohol treatment would be

    Possible ○ ○ ○ ○ ○ ○ ○ Impossible

39. If I wanted to, I could easily go to alcohol treatment.

    Strongly Agree ○ ○ ○ ○ ○ ○ ○ Strongly Disagree

40. Going to alcohol treatment is under my control.

    Completely ○ ○ ○ ○ ○ ○ ○ Not at All

41. I intend to go to alcohol treatment.

    Definitely Yes ○ ○ ○ ○ ○ ○ ○ Definitely Not

42. I will try to go to alcohol treatment.

    Extremely Likely ○ ○ ○ ○ ○ ○ ○ Extremely Unlikely

43. I have decided to go to alcohol treatment.

    Strongly Agree ○ ○ ○ ○ ○ ○ ○ Strongly Disagree

References

Ajzen, I. 1991. "The Theory of Planned Behavior." *Organizational Behavior and Human Decision Processes* 50:179–211.

Beck, J.S. 1995. *Cognitive Therapy: Basics and Beyond.* New York: The Guilford Press.

Craske, M.G. 2004. *Cognitive-Behavioral Treatment of Anxiety Disorders (ACS Manual).* Unpublished reference manual.

Dick, L.P., D. Gallagher-Thompson, D.W. Coon, D.V. Powers, and L.W. Thompson 1996. *Cognitive-Behavioral Therapy for Late-Life Depression: A Therapist Manual.* Palo Alto, CA: Stanford University Press.

Greenberger, D., and C.A. Padesky 2006. *Mind over Mood: Change How You Feel by Changing the Way You Think.* New York: The Guilford Press.

Jaycox, L.H., J. Miranda, L.S. Meredith, N. Duan, B. Benjamin, and K. B. Wells 2003. "Impact of a primary care quality improvement intervention on use of psychotherapy for depression." *Mental Health Services Research* 5(2):109–20.

Muñoz, R.F., C.G. Ippen, S. Rao, H. Le, and E.V. Dwyer 2000. *Manual for Group Cognitive-Behavioral Therapy of Major Depression: A Reality Management Approach—Participant Manual.* San Francisco: University of California, San Francisco University Press.

Padesky, C.A., and D. Greenberger 1995. *Clinician's Guide to Mind over Mood.* New York: The Guilford Press.

Persons, J.B. 1989. *Cognitive Therapy in Practice: A Case Formulation Approach.* New York: W.W. Norton & Company.

Stecker, T., J.C. Fortney, C.D. Sherbourne, and J. Howard 2010. "An intervention to increase mental health treatment engagement among OIF Veterans: A pilot trial." Manuscript submitted for publication.

Unutzer, J. et al. 2002. "Collaborative care management of late-life depression in the primary care setting: A randomized controlled trial." *Journal of the American Medical Association* 288(22):2836–45.

About the Author

Tracy Stecker, Ph.D., is a psychologist and health services researcher at the Psychiatric Research Center at Dartmouth Medical School. Her work focuses on identifying barriers to mental health and substance abuse treatments and developing interventions so that individuals are more likely to access treatment. Her research has been funded by the National Institute of Mental Health, the National Institute of Alcoholism and Alcohol Abuse, and the Department of Veterans Affairs.